Table Of Contents

CHAPTER 1: UNDERSTANDING FASTING FOR WEIGHT LOSS

THE SCIENCE BEHIND FASTING

In the subchapter titled "The Science Behind Fasting," we delve into the physiological processes that occur in the body during a fast. When we abstain from food for an extended period, our bodies enter a state of ketosis, where stored fat is broken down to produce energy. This metabolic state not only aids in weight loss but also has numerous health benefits, such as improved insulin sensitivity and reduced inflammation.

Intermittent fasting is a popular method for weight loss that involves alternating between periods of eating and fasting. By restricting the window of time in which you consume food, you can control your calorie intake and promote fat burning. Studies have shown that intermittent fasting can lead to significant weight loss, particularly around the abdominal area, which is associated with a lower risk of chronic diseases.

For beginners looking to incorporate fasting into their weight loss journey, it is essential to start slowly and gradually increase the duration of fasting periods. Begin by skipping breakfast or delaying your first meal of the day, then progress to longer fasting windows as your body adapts. It is crucial to listen to your body's hunger cues and not push yourself beyond your limits.

Busy professionals often struggle to find time for healthy eating habits, making fasting a convenient option for weight loss. By simplifying meal planning and reducing the number of meals consumed each day, fasting can be a time-saving solution for those with hectic schedules. Additionally, fasting has been shown to improve mental clarity and focus, making it ideal for professionals seeking to enhance their productivity.

Women over 40 may face unique challenges when it comes to losing weight, as hormonal changes can slow down metabolism and lead to stubborn fat accumulation. Fasting can help balance hormone levels and promote weight loss in this demographic. By incorporating fasting into their wellness routine, women over 40 can achieve their weight loss goals and improve overall health.

BENEFITS OF FASTING FOR WEIGHT LOSS

Fasting has been gaining popularity in recent years as a weight loss tool, and for good reason. The benefits of fasting for weight loss are numerous and can be incredibly effective for those looking to shed unwanted pounds. One of the key benefits of fasting for weight loss is its ability to kickstart the body's fat-burning processes. When we fast, our bodies are forced to rely on stored fat for energy, leading to significant weight loss over time.

Another benefit of fasting for weight loss is its ability to regulate hunger hormones. By giving our digestive systems a break through fasting, we can reset our hunger cues and learn to differentiate between true hunger and cravings. This can lead to more mindful eating habits and ultimately, weight loss. Additionally, fasting can help improve insulin sensitivity, making it easier for the body to regulate blood sugar levels and prevent weight gain.

Fasting can also be a powerful tool for improving digestion. By allowing the gut to rest during fasting periods, we can give our digestive systems a chance to repair and heal. This can lead to improved nutrient absorption, reduced bloating and gas, and overall better digestive health. For those struggling with chronic digestive issues, fasting may offer relief and help promote weight loss in the process.

For busy professionals, fasting can be a convenient and time-saving way to lose weight. By simplifying meal planning and reducing the need for constant snacking, fasting can fit seamlessly into a hectic schedule. Additionally, fasting can help improve mental clarity and focus, making it easier to stay productive and on track with weight loss goals. Whether you're a busy executive or a stay-at-home parent, fasting can be a practical and effective weight loss solution.

In conclusion, fasting for weight loss offers a multitude of benefits for those looking to shed excess pounds. From kickstarting fat-burning processes to regulating hunger hormones and improving digestion, fasting can be a powerful tool for achieving weight loss goals. Whether you're a beginner looking to dip your toes into fasting or an experienced faster looking to take your weight loss journey to the next level, incorporating fasting into your routine can lead to lasting results. With the right guidance and a step-by-step approach, you can lose weight, improve your health, and transform your life with fasting.

CHAPTER 2: GETTING STARTED WITH FASTING

CHOOSING THE RIGHT FASTING METHOD

Choosing the right fasting method is crucial when embarking on a journey to lose weight through fasting. With so many different fasting protocols out there, it can be overwhelming to know which one is the best fit for you. It's essential to consider your lifestyle, schedule, health goals, and personal preferences when selecting a fasting method that will work for you.

Intermittent fasting is a popular choice for many people looking to lose weight. This method involves cycling between periods of eating and fasting, typically with a shorter eating window each day. Intermittent fasting can be tailored to fit your schedule, whether you're a busy professional, athlete, or woman over 40. It's important to experiment with different fasting windows to see what works best for your body and lifestyle.

For beginners, starting with a simple fasting method like the 16/8 protocol can be a great way to ease into fasting. This involves fasting for 16 hours each day and eating within an 8-hour window. As you become more comfortable with fasting, you can gradually increase the fasting window or try more advanced fasting methods like alternate day fasting or extended fasting.

When choosing a fasting method, it's essential to consider your goals beyond weight loss. Fasting can have a range of benefits, including improved digestion, mental clarity, hormone balance, and even spiritual growth. If you have specific health conditions, it's important to consult with a healthcare provider before starting any fasting regimen to ensure it's safe and suitable for your individual needs.

Ultimately, the best fasting method is one that you can stick to long-term and that aligns with your health goals and lifestyle. Experiment with different fasting protocols, listen to your body, and make adjustments as needed. Remember that fasting is just one tool in your weight loss journey, and it's important to combine it with a healthy diet, regular exercise, and other lifestyle habits for long-term success.

SETTING REALISTIC GOALS

Setting realistic goals is crucial when embarking on a fasting journey for weight loss. It's important to remember that weight loss is a gradual process and setting achievable goals is key to staying motivated and on track. When setting goals, it's essential to be specific and realistic. For example, instead of saying "I want to lose 30 pounds in a week," a more realistic goal would be "I want to lose 1-2 pounds per week through fasting."

One way to set realistic goals is to break down your ultimate goal into smaller, more manageable milestones. For example, if your goal is to lose 30 pounds, you could set a milestone to lose 5 pounds in the first month. By setting achievable milestones, you can track your progress and celebrate your successes along the way. This can help keep you motivated and focused on your ultimate goal.

Another important aspect of setting realistic goals is to consider your lifestyle and commitments. If you're a busy professional or athlete, it may not be realistic to fast for extended periods of time. Instead, you could try intermittent fasting or shorter fasts that fit into your schedule. By tailoring your fasting plan to your lifestyle, you're more likely to stick with it and see results.

When setting goals, it's also important to consider your overall health and well-being. Fasting can have many benefits beyond weight loss, such as improved digestion, mental clarity, and hormone balance. By setting goals that align with these benefits, you can improve not just your physical appearance, but also your overall health and quality of life.

In conclusion, setting realistic goals is essential when embarking on a fasting journey for weight loss. By being specific, breaking down your ultimate goal into smaller milestones, considering your lifestyle and commitments, and focusing on overall health benefits, you can set yourself up for success. Remember, weight loss is a marathon, not a sprint, and by setting achievable goals, you can stay motivated and on track towards a healthier, happier you.

CHAPTER 3: FASTING FOR BEGINNERS

PREPARING YOUR BODY FOR FASTING

In order to maximize the benefits of fasting for weight loss, it is essential to properly prepare your body beforehand. This subchapter will provide you with valuable tips and techniques to ensure that your body is ready for the fasting process. By following these guidelines, you can make the most out of your fasting journey and achieve your weight loss goals effectively.

First and foremost, it is important to gradually reduce your intake of processed foods, sugars, and caffeine leading up to your fast. This will help to ease your body into the fasting process and reduce any potential withdrawal symptoms. Instead, focus on consuming whole, nutrient-dense foods such as fruits, vegetables, lean proteins, and healthy fats to nourish your body and provide it with the necessary nutrients before fasting.

Hydration is key when preparing for fasting. Make sure to drink plenty of water in the days leading up to your fast to keep your body hydrated and support its detoxification processes. Additionally, herbal teas and electrolyte-rich beverages can help to replenish your body's electrolytes and keep you feeling energized during your fast.

Incorporating light exercise into your routine can also help to prepare your body for fasting. Gentle activities such as yoga, walking, or stretching can improve circulation, reduce stress, and promote relaxation, which can all support your body's ability to fast effectively. Just be sure to listen to your body and avoid high-intensity workouts during this time.

Lastly, mentally preparing yourself for fasting is just as important as physically preparing your body. Take time to set your intentions for the fast, visualize your weight loss goals, and create a positive mindset to support your journey. By approaching fasting with a clear and focused mindset, you can overcome any challenges that may arise and stay committed to achieving your desired results.

OVERCOMING COMMON FASTING CHALLENGES

In the journey of fasting for weight loss, it is common to encounter challenges that may hinder progress and discourage individuals from achieving their goals. However, it is important to remember that these obstacles can be overcome with the right mindset and strategies in place.

One common challenge faced by many individuals when fasting is dealing with hunger pangs and cravings. These feelings can be intense, especially in the beginning stages of fasting. To combat this, it is important to stay hydrated and consume plenty of water throughout the day. Additionally, incorporating healthy fats and protein into meals can help keep you feeling full and satisfied.

Another challenge that individuals may face when fasting is social pressure and temptation. It can be difficult to stick to a fasting regimen when surrounded by friends and family who are not following the same lifestyle. In these situations, it is important to communicate your goals and boundaries to those around you and seek support from like-minded individuals who understand your journey.

One of the biggest challenges when fasting for weight loss is dealing with plateaus. It is common for weight loss to slow down or stall after a period of consistent progress. To overcome this challenge, it is important to reassess your fasting routine and make adjustments as needed. This may include changing up your fasting schedule, incorporating more physical activity, or seeking guidance from a healthcare professional.

Lastly, a common challenge when fasting for weight loss is dealing with negative side effects such as fatigue, dizziness, and mood swings. These symptoms can be a sign that your body is adjusting to the fasting process. To overcome this, it is important to listen to your body and prioritize self-care. Getting plenty of rest, practicing stress-relief techniques, and nourishing your body with nutrient-dense foods can help alleviate these symptoms and support your overall well-being.

By acknowledging and addressing these common fasting challenges, individuals can better navigate their weight loss journey and achieve their goals successfully. Remember that with patience, persistence, and a positive mindset, you can overcome any obstacle that comes your way on the path to achieving a healthier and happier lifestyle through fasting.

CHAPTER 4: INTERMITTENT FASTING FOR WEIGHT LOSS

DIFFERENT INTERMITTENT FASTING METHODS

Intermittent fasting has gained popularity in recent years as a powerful tool for weight loss and overall health. There are several different methods of intermittent fasting, each with its own unique approach and benefits. In this subchapter, we will explore some of the most common intermittent fasting methods and how they can help you achieve your weight loss goals.

One popular method of intermittent fasting is the 16/8 method, where you fast for 16 hours each day and eat all of your meals within an 8-hour window. This method is relatively easy to follow and can be adapted to fit your schedule. By restricting your eating window, you can naturally reduce your calorie intake and promote weight loss.

Another common method is the 5:2 diet, where you eat normally for five days of the week and restrict your calorie intake to 500-600 calories on the other two days. This approach can be effective for weight loss and may also have additional health benefits, such as improved insulin sensitivity and reduced inflammation.

For those looking for a more flexible approach, the eat-stop-eat method involves fasting for 24 hours once or twice a week. This method can be challenging for beginners, but it can be an effective way to kickstart weight loss and improve metabolic health.

The alternate day fasting method involves alternating between days of regular eating and days of fasting. On fasting days, you may consume very few calories or none at all. This method can be effective for weight loss, but it may not be sustainable for everyone in the long term.

Finally, the warrior diet involves fasting for 20 hours each day and eating one large meal in the evening. This method is inspired by the eating patterns of ancient warriors and can be effective for weight loss, improved energy levels, and mental clarity. Experiment with different intermittent fasting methods to find what works best for you and fits your lifestyle. With consistency and dedication, you can achieve your weight loss goals and improve your overall health through intermittent fasting.

HOW INTERMITTENT FASTING CAN HELP YOU LOSE 30 POUNDS

Intermittent fasting has gained popularity in recent years as a powerful tool for weight loss. In this subchapter, we will explore how intermittent fasting can help you lose 30 pounds and achieve your weight loss goals. By following a step-by-step guide to fasting for weight loss, you can see significant results in a relatively short amount of time.

Intermittent fasting involves cycling between periods of eating and fasting, with the goal of reducing overall calorie intake and promoting fat loss. This approach has been shown to be effective for weight loss, as it can help regulate hormones that control appetite and metabolism. By following a daily guide to fasting, you can establish a routine that works for your lifestyle and goals.

For beginners, intermittent fasting may seem daunting at first. However, with the right approach and mindset, you can easily incorporate fasting into your daily routine. By gradually increasing the length of your fasting periods and adjusting your eating habits, you can train your body to burn fat for energy and see the pounds melt away.

Busy professionals, women over 40, athletes, and individuals with chronic health conditions can all benefit from intermittent fasting. Not only does fasting help with weight loss, but it can also improve digestion, promote mental clarity, balance hormones, and even support spiritual growth. By making fasting a part of your daily routine, you can experience a wide range of health benefits beyond just losing weight.

In conclusion, intermittent fasting is a powerful tool for weight loss that can help you shed 30 pounds and achieve your desired physique. By following a step-by-step guide to fasting, you can establish a sustainable routine that works for your lifestyle and goals. Whether you are a beginner or an experienced faster, incorporating fasting into your daily routine can lead to significant improvements in your overall health and well-being.

CHAPTER 5: FASTING FOR BUSY PROFESSIONALS

INCORPORATING FASTING INTO A BUSY SCHEDULE

Incorporating fasting into a busy schedule can seem like a daunting task, especially for those with hectic lifestyles. However, with proper planning and dedication, it is entirely possible to successfully integrate fasting into your daily routine. By following a few simple tips and tricks, you can make fasting a seamless part of your weight loss journey.

One of the key strategies for incorporating fasting into a busy schedule is to plan ahead. Take some time each week to map out your fasting schedule, including when you will be eating and when you will be fasting. By having a clear plan in place, you can ensure that you stay on track and avoid any unnecessary pitfalls that may derail your progress.

Another important aspect of incorporating fasting into a busy schedule is to be flexible. Life can be unpredictable, and there may be days when fasting is simply not feasible. Instead of getting discouraged, try to adjust your fasting schedule to accommodate these unexpected events. Remember, consistency is key when it comes to fasting for weight loss, so do your best to stay on track even when faced with challenges.

For busy professionals, finding time to fast can be especially challenging. However, with a bit of creativity, it is possible to make fasting work within even the most demanding work schedules. Consider fasting during your commute to work, or during meetings when you know you won't be eating anyway. By finding pockets of time throughout your day to fast, you can stay on track with your weight loss goals without sacrificing your professional responsibilities.

Incorporating fasting into a busy schedule is not just about weight loss – it can also have a positive impact on your mental clarity, digestion, hormone balance, and overall health. By taking the time to prioritize fasting in your daily routine, you can experience a wide range of benefits that go beyond just shedding pounds. Whether you are a busy professional, an athlete, a woman over 40, or someone managing chronic health conditions, fasting can be a powerful tool for improving your overall well-being. So don't let a hectic schedule stand in the way of your weight loss goals – with a bit of planning and dedication, you can successfully incorporate fasting into your busy life and achieve the results you desire.

TIPS FOR FASTING AT WORK

Fasting at work can be a challenge, especially for those who have busy schedules and demanding jobs. However, with the right tips and strategies, it is possible to successfully fast while at work and continue on the path to weight loss and improved health. Here are some helpful tips for fasting at work:

1. Plan ahead: Before starting your fast, take some time to plan out your meals and snacks for the day. Bring pre-portioned, healthy snacks like nuts, seeds, fruits, and vegetables to keep you satisfied and energized throughout the day. Make sure to also have plenty of water on hand to stay hydrated and ward off hunger cravings.

2. Schedule your fast strategically: If possible, try to schedule your fast during times when you have fewer work commitments or meetings. This will help you avoid distractions and stay focused on your fasting goals. Consider starting your fast after lunch or in the evening to make it easier to resist temptations during the workday.

3. Stay busy: Keep yourself occupied during your fasting period to avoid thinking about food or feeling hungry. Stay focused on your work tasks, take short breaks to go for a walk or stretch, or engage in a quiet activity like reading or meditating. Keeping your mind busy will help you stay on track with your fasting goals.

4. Communicate with coworkers: Let your coworkers know that you are fasting so they can support you in your efforts. Avoid office gatherings or events that involve food during your fasting period, and politely decline any offers of snacks or meals. Having the support of your colleagues can make fasting at work easier and more manageable.

5. Listen to your body: Pay attention to how you are feeling during your fast and adjust accordingly. If you are feeling lightheaded, dizzy, or weak, it may be a sign that you need to break your fast and eat a small, healthy meal. Remember, fasting should not be a punishment, but a tool to improve your health and well-being. Listen to your body and prioritize your health above all else. With these tips in mind, you can successfully fast at work and continue on your journey to losing weight and achieving your health goals.

CHAPTER 6: FASTING FOR WOMEN OVER 40

HORMONAL CHANGES AND FASTING

When it comes to losing weight, understanding the role of hormones in our body is crucial. Hormones play a key role in regulating our metabolism, hunger levels, and overall energy balance. Fasting can have a significant impact on our hormones, leading to positive changes that can aid in weight loss.

One of the main hormones affected by fasting is insulin. Insulin is responsible for regulating blood sugar levels and storing excess energy as fat. When we fast, insulin levels decrease, allowing our body to burn stored fat for energy instead of relying on glucose. This can lead to accelerated fat loss and improved metabolic health.

Another hormone that is affected by fasting is ghrelin, also known as the hunger hormone. Ghrelin is responsible for signaling hunger to the brain. When we fast, ghrelin levels initially increase, causing hunger pangs. However, over time, ghrelin levels tend to decrease, leading to reduced feelings of hunger and increased satiety. This can make it easier to stick to a fasting regimen and consume fewer calories overall.

In addition to insulin and ghrelin, fasting can also impact other hormones such as growth hormone and cortisol. Growth hormone is essential for fat loss and muscle growth, and fasting can increase its production. Cortisol, on the other hand, is known as the stress hormone and can be elevated in response to prolonged fasting. It is important to manage stress levels and ensure adequate rest during fasting to prevent negative effects on cortisol levels.

For women over 40, hormonal changes can play a significant role in weight loss and fasting. As women age, estrogen levels decrease, leading to changes in metabolism and fat distribution. Fasting can help balance hormones and improve metabolic health in women over 40, leading to more effective weight loss results. It is important for women in this age group to consult with a healthcare provider before starting a fasting regimen to ensure it is safe and appropriate for their individual needs.

In conclusion, understanding the hormonal changes that occur during fasting is essential for successful weight loss. By harnessing the power of hormones such as insulin, ghrelin, growth hormone, and cortisol, fasting can be a powerful tool for achieving your weight loss goals. Whether you are a beginner to fasting or a seasoned pro, incorporating fasting into your routine can lead to improved digestion, mental clarity, hormone balance, and overall health. Remember to listen to your body, stay hydrated, and prioritize self-care to maximize the benefits of fasting for weight loss.

FASTING SAFELY AS A WOMAN OVER 40

Fasting can be a powerful tool for weight loss, but for women over 40, it's essential to approach fasting with caution and mindfulness. As our bodies age, our metabolism slows down and hormonal changes can impact how we respond to fasting. By following these tips, you can fast safely and effectively to support your weight loss goals.

First and foremost, it's crucial to listen to your body and pay attention to how you feel during the fasting process. Women over 40 may have different nutritional needs than younger individuals, so it's important to tailor your fasting plan to suit your unique requirements. If you experience any negative side effects such as dizziness, fatigue, or extreme hunger, it may be a sign that you need to adjust your fasting schedule or seek guidance from a healthcare professional.

When fasting as a woman over 40, it's also important to prioritize nutrient-dense foods during your eating windows. Focus on consuming plenty of lean protein, healthy fats, fruits, vegetables, and whole grains to support your overall health and well-being. Avoid processed foods, sugary snacks, and excessive caffeine, as these can disrupt your hormonal balance and hinder your weight loss progress.

Intermittent fasting is a popular approach for women over 40 looking to lose weight, as it allows for flexibility in your eating patterns while still promoting fat loss. Consider starting with a 16:8 fasting schedule, where you fast for 16 hours and eat within an 8-hour window each day. This can help regulate your blood sugar levels, improve insulin sensitivity, and promote fat burning, all of which are key factors in successful weight loss.

In addition to weight loss, fasting can also offer a range of other health benefits for women over 40, including improved digestion, hormone balance, mental clarity, and even spiritual growth. By incorporating fasting into your routine mindfully and safely, you can unlock the full potential of this powerful tool for transforming your health and achieving your weight loss goals. Remember to consult with a healthcare provider before starting any fasting regimen, especially if you have underlying health conditions or concerns.

CHAPTER 7: FASTING FOR ATHLETES

FUELING YOUR WORKOUTS WITH FASTING

When it comes to losing weight and achieving your fitness goals, fueling your workouts is essential. Many people believe that fasting means depriving your body of the nutrients it needs to exercise effectively. However, when done correctly, fasting can actually enhance your workouts and help you achieve your weight loss goals faster.

Intermittent fasting is a popular method for weight loss that involves cycling between periods of eating and fasting. By incorporating fasting into your workout routine, you can tap into your body's stored fat for energy, leading to more efficient fat burning during exercise. This can help you lose weight faster and improve your overall fitness levels.

For beginners looking to incorporate fasting into their workout routine, it's important to start slowly and listen to your body. Begin by gradually increasing the length of your fasting periods and monitoring how your body responds during workouts. It's also important to stay hydrated and replenish your electrolytes during fasting periods to ensure you have enough energy for exercise.

Busy professionals and athletes can benefit from fasting by scheduling their workouts during fasting periods when their bodies are already in a fat-burning state. This can help maximize the benefits of fasting for weight loss and improve athletic performance. Additionally, fasting can help improve mental clarity and focus, making it easier to stay motivated and committed to your fitness goals.

Women over 40 may find fasting to be particularly beneficial for weight loss, hormone balance, and managing chronic health conditions. Fasting can help regulate insulin levels, reduce inflammation, and improve digestion, all of which can contribute to long-term weight loss and overall well-being. By incorporating fasting into your routine, you can take control of your health and achieve your weight loss goals in a sustainable way.

In conclusion, fueling your workouts with fasting can be a powerful tool for weight loss and overall wellness. By incorporating fasting into your routine, you can tap into your body's natural fat-burning abilities, improve your fitness levels, and achieve your weight loss goals faster. Whether you're a beginner or an experienced faster, there are many ways to incorporate fasting into your workout routine and take control of your health.

RECOVERING FROM EXERCISE WHILE FASTING

One of the key components of a successful weight loss journey through fasting is incorporating exercise into your routine. However, when you are fasting, it is important to pay special attention to how you recover from your workouts to ensure that you are not putting unnecessary strain on your body. Here are some tips for recovering from exercise while fasting.

First and foremost, it is essential to listen to your body. If you are feeling extremely fatigued or sore after a workout while fasting, it may be a sign that you need to dial back the intensity or duration of your exercise routine. Fasting can put additional stress on your body, so it is important to give yourself permission to take it easy when needed.

Hydration is key when recovering from exercise while fasting. Since you are not consuming food during your fasting period, it is even more important to make sure you are drinking enough water to replenish the fluids lost during your workout. You may also consider adding some electrolytes to your water to help replace any lost minerals.

Incorporating a post-workout meal or snack into your fasting routine can also help with recovery. While you may not be breaking your fast right after your workout, having a nutritious meal or snack ready to go can help replenish your energy stores and aid in muscle recovery. Consider including protein and healthy fats in your post-workout meal to help repair and build muscle.

Getting an adequate amount of rest is crucial for recovery, especially when fasting. Your body needs time to repair and rebuild muscle tissue, so make sure you are giving yourself enough time to rest and recover between workouts. Aim for at least 7-8 hours of quality sleep each night to support your weight loss goals.

Lastly, consider incorporating some gentle stretching or yoga into your routine to help with recovery while fasting. Stretching can help improve flexibility, reduce muscle soreness, and promote relaxation. It can also help improve circulation and aid in the removal of waste products from your muscles, helping you recover more quickly from your workouts.

CHAPTER 8: FASTING FOR MENTAL CLARITY

HOW FASTING CAN IMPROVE COGNITIVE FUNCTION

Fasting is not just a tool for weight loss, but it can also greatly improve cognitive function. When we fast, our bodies switch from using glucose as a primary fuel source to using ketones, which are produced from stored fat. This shift can lead to increased mental clarity, focus, and concentration. Many people report feeling more alert and productive during fasting periods, making it an ideal practice for busy professionals looking to optimize their work performance.

Intermittent fasting, in particular, has been shown to have numerous cognitive benefits. By incorporating regular fasting periods into your daily routine, you can improve brain function, memory, and mood. This is because fasting helps to reduce inflammation in the brain, which is linked to cognitive decline and neurodegenerative diseases. For those looking to boost their mental clarity and overall brain health, intermittent fasting can be a powerful tool.

Women over 40 may also benefit from fasting when it comes to cognitive function. As we age, our brains can become more susceptible to cognitive decline and memory loss. By incorporating fasting into their routine, women over 40 can help protect their brain health and improve cognitive function. Fasting has been shown to promote the growth of new brain cells and enhance synaptic plasticity, which is crucial for learning and memory.

Athletes can also benefit from fasting when it comes to cognitive function. By training in a fasted state, athletes can enhance their mental focus and endurance. Fasting helps to increase the production of brain-derived neurotrophic factor (BDNF), a protein that supports the growth and survival of neurons. This can lead to improved cognitive function, better decision-making skills, and enhanced athletic performance.

In conclusion, fasting is not just a powerful tool for weight loss, but it can also significantly improve cognitive function. Whether you are a busy professional looking to boost your productivity, a woman over 40 wanting to protect your brain health, or an athlete seeking to enhance your mental focus, incorporating fasting into your routine can have numerous cognitive benefits. By fueling your body with ketones and reducing inflammation in the brain, fasting can lead to increased mental clarity, focus, and overall brain health.

TIPS FOR FASTING TO BOOST MENTAL CLARITY

Fasting is not only a great way to shed extra pounds, but it can also have a profound effect on your mental clarity. When done correctly, fasting can help improve focus, concentration, and overall cognitive function. Here are some tips for fasting to boost mental clarity:

1. Stay hydrated: One of the most important aspects of fasting is to stay hydrated. Dehydration can lead to brain fog and lack of focus, so be sure to drink plenty of water throughout the day. Herbal teas and black coffee are also great options to help keep you hydrated while fasting.

2. Get plenty of rest: Fasting can be taxing on the body, so it's important to get plenty of rest during this time. Make sure to prioritize sleep and listen to your body when it's telling you to rest. Adequate rest will help improve mental clarity and overall well-being.

3. Practice mindfulness: Fasting can be a great opportunity to practice mindfulness and focus on the present moment. Take time each day to meditate, practice deep breathing exercises, or simply sit quietly and reflect on your goals. This can help reduce stress and improve mental clarity during your fasting period.

4. Stay active: Regular exercise is not only important for weight loss, but it can also help boost mental clarity. Even a short walk or yoga session can help improve focus and concentration. Find an activity that you enjoy and make it a priority during your fasting period.

5. Break your fast with nutrient-dense foods: When it's time to break your fast, opt for nutrient-dense foods that will help nourish your body and brain. Include plenty of fruits, vegetables, lean proteins, and healthy fats in your meals to help fuel your body and improve mental clarity. Avoid processed foods and sugary treats, as these can lead to energy crashes and brain fog. By following these tips, you can make the most of your fasting period and experience improved mental clarity along with your weight loss goals.

CHAPTER 9: FASTING FOR IMPROVED DIGESTION

HEALING YOUR GUT THROUGH FASTING

In the journey to weight loss, many people overlook the importance of healing their gut through fasting. Fasting can be a powerful tool in improving digestion and overall gut health. By giving your digestive system a break from constant food intake, you allow it time to repair and reset. This can lead to improved nutrient absorption, reduced inflammation, and a healthier gut microbiome.

Intermittent fasting, in particular, has been shown to have numerous benefits for gut health. By cycling between periods of eating and fasting, you give your gut a chance to rest and recover. This can help reduce symptoms of bloating, gas, and indigestion, as well as improve overall gut function. Intermittent fasting can also help regulate hormone levels that play a role in digestion, such as insulin and ghrelin.

For beginners looking to incorporate fasting into their weight loss journey, it's important to start slow and listen to your body. Begin with shorter fasting windows, such as 12-14 hours, and gradually increase the length as you become more comfortable. It's also important to stay hydrated and nourish your body with nutrient-dense foods during your eating window to support gut health.

Busy professionals may find fasting to be a convenient way to support weight loss and improve digestion. With a busy schedule, fasting can simplify meal planning and reduce the need for constant snacking. By incorporating fasting into your routine, you can boost energy levels, improve mental clarity, and support overall gut health.

In conclusion, healing your gut through fasting can be a powerful tool in achieving weight loss goals. Whether you're looking to lose 30 pounds or simply improve your digestion, fasting can support your journey. By incorporating intermittent fasting into your routine and listening to your body's cues, you can experience the numerous benefits of fasting for improved gut health and overall well-being.

FOODS TO BREAK YOUR FAST FOR BETTER DIGESTION

Breaking your fast with the right foods can make a big difference in how your body digests and absorbs nutrients. When you have been fasting for an extended period, it's important to reintroduce food in a gentle and nurturing way to avoid overwhelming your digestive system. Here are some foods that can help you break your fast for better digestion.

One of the best foods to break your fast with is bone broth. Bone broth is rich in nutrients and minerals that are easily absorbed by the body. It also contains gelatin and collagen, which can help to heal and seal the gut lining, improving digestion. Start your day with a warm cup of bone broth to kickstart your digestive system and provide your body with essential nutrients.

Another great option for breaking your fast is fermented foods, such as sauerkraut or kimchi. Fermented foods are rich in probiotics, which are beneficial bacteria that support gut health and aid in digestion. Adding fermented foods to your first meal of the day can help to replenish the good bacteria in your gut and improve overall digestive function.

Fruits are also a good choice for breaking your fast, as they are easy to digest and provide a quick source of energy. Opt for low-glycemic fruits like berries, apples, or pears to avoid spiking your blood sugar levels. Fruits are also rich in fiber, which can help to regulate digestion and promote a healthy gut microbiome.

Leafy greens are another excellent option for breaking your fast. Greens like spinach, kale, and arugula are packed with vitamins, minerals, and antioxidants that support overall digestive health. They are also high in fiber, which can help to promote regular bowel movements and prevent constipation. Incorporate a serving of leafy greens into your first meal of the day to support optimal digestion.

Finally, don't forget to drink plenty of water throughout the day to stay hydrated and support digestion. Water helps to flush out toxins, aid in nutrient absorption, and keep your digestive system functioning properly. Aim to drink at least 8-10 glasses of water each day, and consider adding lemon or cucumber slices for added flavor and digestion-boosting benefits. By choosing the right foods to break your fast, you can support better digestion and overall health on your weight loss journey.

CHAPTER 10: FASTING FOR SPIRITUAL GROWTH

USING FASTING AS A SPIRITUAL PRACTICE

Using fasting as a spiritual practice can be a powerful tool for those looking to lose weight and improve their overall well-being. Fasting has been used for centuries by various cultures and religions as a way to cleanse the body and mind, and to connect with something greater than ourselves. By incorporating fasting into your weight loss journey, you can not only shed those extra pounds but also cultivate a deeper sense of self-awareness and mindfulness.

When you fast, you are giving your body a break from constantly digesting food, allowing it to focus on healing and rejuvenating itself. This can lead to increased energy levels, improved digestion, and a clearer mind. By using fasting as a spiritual practice, you can take this time to reflect on your goals, motivations, and values, and gain a deeper understanding of yourself and your relationship with food.

For those who are new to fasting, it is important to start slow and gradually build up your fasting duration. Intermittent fasting, where you restrict your eating window to a set number of hours each day, is a great way to ease into fasting and still experience its benefits. By following a step-by-step daily guide, you can learn how to incorporate fasting into your routine in a safe and sustainable way.

Fasting can be especially beneficial for busy professionals who are looking to lose weight but struggle to find the time for traditional diet and exercise routines. By incorporating fasting into your daily schedule, you can simplify your eating habits and focus on nourishing your body with whole, nutrient-dense foods during your eating window. This can lead to improved digestion, increased energy levels, and better overall health.

In addition to the physical benefits of fasting, many people also find that it can help them achieve a deeper sense of spiritual growth and connection. By using fasting as a way to practice mindfulness and self-discipline, you can cultivate a greater sense of gratitude, compassion, and inner peace. Whether you are fasting for weight loss, improved digestion, hormone balance, or mental clarity, incorporating a spiritual aspect into your fasting practice can help you stay motivated and inspired on your journey to better health and well-being.

CONNECTING MIND, BODY, AND SPIRIT THROUGH FASTING

In this subchapter, we will explore the powerful connection between the mind, body, and spirit through the practice of fasting for weight loss. Fasting is not just about restricting food intake, but rather a holistic approach to wellness that can transform your entire being.

When we fast, we are not only giving our bodies a break from digesting food, but we are also giving our minds a chance to reset and rejuvenate. Fasting allows us to focus inward, to reflect on our goals and intentions, and to cultivate a sense of mindfulness and awareness that can help us make healthier choices in all areas of our lives.

Connecting the mind, body, and spirit through fasting can lead to a deeper sense of self-awareness and self-control. By tuning into our bodies' signals and listening to what they truly need, we can break free from emotional eating patterns and develop a healthier relationship with food.

Fasting can also be a powerful tool for spiritual growth and connection. Many cultures and religions have long embraced fasting as a way to cleanse the body and soul, and to deepen one's connection to the divine. By incorporating fasting into your weight loss journey, you can tap into a deeper sense of purpose and meaning, and find strength and guidance from within.

In conclusion, fasting is not just a physical practice, but a mental, emotional, and spiritual one as well. By connecting mind, body, and spirit through fasting for weight loss, you can achieve not only a slimmer waistline, but also a greater sense of well-being and fulfillment in all areas of your life. So, as you embark on your fasting journey, remember to nourish not just your body, but your mind and spirit as well.

CHAPTER 11: FASTING FOR HORMONE BALANCE

BALANCING HORMONES THROUGH FASTING

When it comes to losing weight, many people focus solely on diet and exercise, but one key component that often gets overlooked is hormone balance. Hormones play a crucial role in regulating our metabolism, hunger levels, and energy levels, making them a crucial factor in achieving weight loss goals. One powerful way to balance hormones and support weight loss is through fasting.

Fasting has been shown to have a positive impact on hormone levels, particularly insulin and leptin. Insulin is the hormone responsible for regulating blood sugar levels and storing fat, while leptin is the hormone that signals to the brain that we are full. By incorporating fasting into your weight loss journey, you can help regulate these hormones and promote a healthier metabolism.

One of the main ways that fasting helps balance hormones is by reducing insulin resistance. When we fast, our body is forced to use stored fat for energy, which can help decrease insulin levels and improve insulin sensitivity. This can lead to better blood sugar control and a more efficient metabolism, making weight loss easier and more sustainable in the long run.

In addition to insulin, fasting can also help regulate leptin levels. Leptin resistance is common in overweight individuals, leading to increased hunger and decreased feelings of fullness. By incorporating fasting into your routine, you can help reset your leptin sensitivity and improve your body's ability to regulate hunger and satiety, making it easier to stick to a healthy eating plan and avoid overeating.

Overall, fasting can be a powerful tool for balancing hormones and supporting weight loss. By incorporating fasting into your routine, you can help regulate insulin and leptin levels, improve metabolism, and support sustainable weight loss goals. Whether you're a busy professional, athlete, or someone looking to improve their overall health, fasting can be a valuable tool for achieving your weight loss goals and improving hormone balance.

MANAGING MENOPAUSE SYMPTOMS WITH FASTING

Menopause is a natural phase in a woman's life that marks the end of her reproductive years. However, it often comes with a host of unpleasant symptoms such as hot flashes, mood swings, and weight gain. Fasting can be a powerful tool for managing these symptoms and improving overall well-being during this transitional phase.

Intermittent fasting, in particular, has been shown to be effective in reducing menopausal symptoms. By restricting the window of time in which you eat, you can regulate hormone levels and reduce inflammation in the body. This can help alleviate hot flashes and mood swings, as well as promote weight loss.

For women over 40 who are experiencing menopause, fasting can be a game-changer. Not only can it help with weight loss, but it can also improve digestion and support hormone balance. By giving your body a break from constant eating, you allow it to repair and regenerate, leading to overall better health and well-being.

Busy professionals who are juggling work, family, and other responsibilities may find fasting to be a convenient way to manage menopause symptoms. With a step-by-step daily guide, you can easily incorporate fasting into your routine without feeling overwhelmed. Plus, the mental clarity and increased energy that come with fasting can help you stay focused and productive throughout the day.

Athletes, too, can benefit from fasting during menopause. By optimizing hormone balance and reducing inflammation, fasting can improve performance and recovery. Whether you're training for a marathon or simply trying to stay active, fasting can help support your fitness goals and overall well-being.

In conclusion, fasting is a powerful tool for managing menopause symptoms and improving overall health during this transitional phase. Whether you're looking to lose weight, balance hormones, or improve digestion, fasting can help you achieve your goals. By following a step-by-step guide and incorporating fasting into your daily routine, you can experience the many benefits that fasting has to offer.

CHAPTER 12: FASTING FOR MANAGING CHRONIC HEALTH CONDITIONS

FASTING FOR DIABETES MANAGEMENT

Fasting can be a powerful tool for managing diabetes and improving overall health. For people wanting to lose weight and improve their insulin sensitivity, fasting can be a game-changer. By giving your body a break from constant food intake, you can help regulate blood sugar levels and reduce the risk of complications associated with diabetes.

Intermittent fasting, in particular, has been shown to be effective for weight loss and improving insulin sensitivity. By alternating between periods of eating and fasting, you can help regulate blood sugar levels and reduce inflammation in the body. This can lead to better overall health and a reduced risk of developing diabetes-related complications.

For beginners looking to incorporate fasting into their routine, it's important to start slow and gradually increase the duration of your fasts. Begin by skipping breakfast and gradually extend the fasting window to 16-18 hours. This can help your body adjust to the new eating pattern and prevent any negative side effects.

Busy professionals may find it challenging to incorporate fasting into their busy schedules, but with some planning and preparation, it is possible. By meal prepping and choosing convenient fasting methods like the 16/8 method, you can easily fit fasting into your daily routine. This can help you achieve your weight loss goals and improve your overall health without sacrificing productivity.

Women over 40 may find that fasting can help manage hormonal imbalances and improve insulin sensitivity. By incorporating fasting into their routine, women can reduce the risk of developing diabetes and other chronic health conditions. With the guidance of a healthcare professional, fasting can be a safe and effective tool for managing diabetes and improving overall health.

USING FASTING TO IMPROVE HEART HEALTH

Fasting has been used for centuries as a way to improve overall health and well-being. One of the many benefits of fasting is its ability to improve heart health. By abstaining from food for a period of time, you give your heart a much-needed break from constantly digesting and processing food. This break allows your heart to work more efficiently and can lead to a decrease in blood pressure and cholesterol levels.

Intermittent fasting is a popular method for using fasting to improve heart health. By cycling between periods of eating and fasting, you can help regulate your blood sugar levels and reduce inflammation in the body, both of which are key factors in maintaining a healthy heart. Intermittent fasting has also been shown to improve insulin sensitivity, which can help prevent heart disease and other chronic conditions.

For those looking to improve their heart health through fasting, it is important to start slowly and gradually increase the length of your fasting periods. Begin by fasting for 12-16 hours overnight and gradually work your way up to longer fasts of 24 hours or more. It is also important to stay hydrated during fasting periods and listen to your body's signals to ensure you are not overdoing it.

Fasting can be particularly beneficial for busy professionals who may not have time to prepare healthy meals or fit in regular exercise. By incorporating fasting into their routine, they can still reap the benefits of improved heart health without the need for strict dieting or intense workout regimens. Fasting can also be a great option for athletes looking to improve their performance, as it can help increase fat burning and improve overall energy levels.

In conclusion, using fasting to improve heart health can be a powerful tool for those looking to lose weight and improve their overall well-being. By incorporating fasting into your routine, you can help regulate blood sugar levels, reduce inflammation, and improve insulin sensitivity, all of which are key factors in maintaining a healthy heart. Whether you are a beginner looking to try fasting for the first time or a busy professional looking for a convenient way to improve your health, fasting can be a valuable tool for achieving your weight loss goals and improving your heart health.

CONCLUSION: ACHIEVING YOUR WEIGHT LOSS GOALS WITH FASTING

In conclusion, achieving your weight loss goals with fasting is not only possible but also incredibly effective. By following the step-by-step guide outlined in this book, you can lose up to 30 pounds and more through fasting. Whether you are new to fasting or a seasoned veteran, the strategies and tips provided can help you reach your desired weight in a healthy and sustainable way.

Intermittent fasting has been shown to be an excellent tool for weight loss, as it allows you to control your calorie intake and improve your metabolism. By incorporating fasting into your daily routine, you can see significant changes in your body composition and overall health. This method is especially beneficial for busy professionals and women over 40 who may struggle to find time for traditional diets and exercise routines.

For athletes looking to improve their performance, fasting can be a game-changer. By utilizing fasting protocols, athletes can optimize their energy levels, improve their endurance, and enhance their recovery time. Fasting can also help athletes maintain a healthy weight and body composition, leading to better results on the field or in the gym.

In addition to weight loss, fasting can also provide mental clarity, improved digestion, hormone balance, and even spiritual growth. Many people find that fasting helps them to focus better, think more clearly, and feel more connected to their bodies and minds. By incorporating fasting into your life, you can experience a range of physical, mental, and emotional benefits that go beyond just losing weight.

Overall, fasting is a powerful tool that can help you achieve your weight loss goals and improve your overall health and well-being. By following the advice and strategies outlined in this book, you can embark on a fasting journey that will transform your body, mind, and spirit. Whether you are looking to lose weight, improve your athletic performance, or simply feel better in your own skin, fasting can be the key to unlocking your full potential.

www.ingramcontent.com/pod-product-compliance
Lightning Source LLC
Chambersburg PA
CBHW081545250726
48659CB00009B/3090